I0843944

Contents

Abstract

"Rapid Weight Loss: A Comprehensive Guide to Transformative Results" is an in-depth exploration of effective strategies for achieving rapid and sustainable weight loss. This ebook guides readers through a holistic approach, encompassing dietary modifications, exercise routines, lifestyle adjustments, and psychological considerations.

The journey begins with an honest assessment of the current lifestyle, prompting readers to analyze their dietary habits, exercise routines, and potential contributors to weight gain. Practical tips and evidence-based strategies are provided to initiate meaningful changes.

The subsequent chapters delve into creating a strategic meal plan, incorporating effective exercises, optimizing hydration and detoxification, and addressing crucial factors like sleep, stress, and supplementation. Each chapter offers detailed insights, practical tips, and evidence-backed recommendations to empower readers on their weight loss journey.

Special emphasis is placed on the importance of setting measurable goals, monitoring progress, and adapting plans to ensure sustained success. The ebook concludes by guiding readers on the transition from intense weight loss efforts to a balanced, long-term lifestyle that promotes physical and mental well-being.

Overall, this comprehensive guide is a roadmap for those seeking not only rapid weight loss but also sustainable health transformations. It encourages readers to approach their journey with a balanced mindset, prioritize well-being, and embrace a holistic lifestyle for enduring success.

Introduction

In a world where time seems to move faster than ever, the desire for swift and effective solutions to weight loss has become a common pursuit. This ebook, "Rapid Weight Loss: A Practical Guide to Shedding Pounds in Days," aims to be your comprehensive companion on a journey towards achieving noticeable and sustainable weight loss within a condensed timeframe.

Before we embark on this transformative expedition, it is crucial to approach it with a balanced mindset. Rapid weight loss is a nuanced process that encompasses various elements, including dietary adjustments, increased physical activity, and lifestyle modifications. While the goal is to witness tangible changes in a short span, it is equally important to prioritize health, well-being, and long-term sustainability.

Within the pages of this guide, we will navigate the intricacies of rapid weight loss, offering not just quick fixes but a holistic approach that considers your overall health. It is essential to understand that each individual's body is unique, responding differently to various methods. This guide is designed to empower you with practical tips, evidence-based strategies, and a realistic perspective on achieving your weight loss goals efficiently.

However, always keep in mind that your health is paramount. Before making significant changes to your diet, exercise routine, or lifestyle, it is advisable to consult with a healthcare professional. This ensures that your journey towards rapid weight loss is not just effective but also safe and tailored to your specific needs.

Now, let's embark on this transformative path together, armed with knowledge, determination, and a commitment to not just losing weight quickly, but to a healthier and more vibrant version of yourself.

Chapter One

Assess Your Current Lifestyle

Embarking on the journey towards rapid weight loss necessitates a comprehensive evaluation of your current lifestyle. The intricacies of daily habits, dietary choices, and physical activity levels all play pivotal roles in the quest for shedding pounds effectively. In this chapter, we will delve into each of these aspects, offering a nuanced understanding and practical strategies to initiate transformative changes.

Analyzing Your Diet

Begin by conducting a thorough analysis of your dietary habits. It's not just about counting calories; it's about understanding the quality of the calories you consume. Take note of the types of foods dominating your plate—Are there too many processed and sugary items? Identifying and addressing these dietary patterns is fundamental to cultivating a more balanced and nourishing approach to eating.

Consider incorporating more nutrient-dense foods into your meals, such as fruits, vegetables, lean proteins, and whole grains. Opt for complex carbohydrates over refined ones and choose sources of healthy fats, like avocados and nuts. Small, mindful changes to your diet can have a profound impact on your overall health and contribute significantly to your weight loss goals.

Evaluating Physical Activity Levels

Physical activity is a cornerstone of any successful weight loss journey. Assess your current exercise routine, if one exists. Are you engaging in regular physical activity, or does a sedentary lifestyle prevail? Recognizing and acknowledging your baseline activity levels is the first step towards establishing a foundation for a more active and health-oriented lifestyle.

Consider incorporating both cardiovascular exercises and strength training into your routine. Cardiovascular activities, such as brisk walking, jogging, or cycling, elevate your heart rate and burn calories, while strength training helps build lean muscle mass, which can boost your metabolism. Finding activities you enjoy can make the process more sustainable and enjoyable.

Identifying Habits that Contribute to Weight Gain

Beyond diet and exercise, it's crucial to delve into the habits that may be impeding your weight loss progress. Late-night snacking, emotional eating, or erratic sleep patterns can significantly impact your ability to shed pounds rapidly. Identifying these habits requires a degree of self-awareness and a commitment to positive change.

Developing healthier alternatives to cope with stress or emotions, creating a consistent sleep schedule, and being mindful of portion sizes are all essential steps in addressing these habits. Recognizing the triggers that lead to unhealthy behaviors empowers you to make informed decisions and cultivate a more supportive environment for your weight loss goals.

As we navigate through the intricacies of analyzing your current lifestyle, keep in mind that the objective is not just to make temporary changes but to lay the groundwork for sustainable and lasting transformation. Assess where you are, envision where you want to be, and let's embark on this journey towards a healthier, more vibrant version of yourself.

Chapter Two

Creating a Strategic Meal Plan

In the intricate tapestry of rapid weight loss, a strategic and well-balanced meal plan emerges as a cornerstone for success. This chapter aims to guide you through the art of making conscious and informed choices about the foods you consume, emphasizing nutrient-rich options and optimal meal timing to amplify the effectiveness of your weight loss endeavors.

Choosing Nutrient-Rich Foods

The heart of any effective meal plan lies in the meticulous selection of foods that offer maximum nutritional value without an excess of calories. It's not just about counting calories but about ensuring that each morsel contributes to your overall well-being. Consider incorporating a vibrant array of fruits and vegetables into your daily meals, embracing their diverse spectrum of vitamins, minerals, and antioxidants.

Lean proteins, derived from sources such as chicken, fish, legumes, and tofu, play a pivotal role in maintaining muscle mass while contributing to a feeling of satiety. Whole grains, like brown rice and quinoa, introduce complex carbohydrates into your diet, providing sustained energy and essential fiber for digestive health. And let's not forget the significance of healthy fats—avocados, nuts, and olive oil offer a wealth of nutrients, supporting everything from brain function to nutrient absorption.

Incorporating Whole Grains, Lean Proteins, and Healthy Fats

Striking the right balance between these three macronutrients is crucial for crafting a meal plan that not only facilitates rapid weight loss but also promotes overall health. Experiment with different combinations and recipes to keep your meals exciting and satisfying.

Whole Grains: The inclusion of whole grains provides a valuable source of fiber, promoting digestive health and helping control appetite. Explore a variety of options, such as quinoa, brown rice, oats, and whole-grain bread, to diversify your nutrient intake.

Lean Proteins: Essential for maintaining muscle mass, lean proteins also contribute to a prolonged feeling of fullness. Consider incorporating poultry, fish, legumes, and plant-based protein sources into your meals. Experiment with different cooking methods and flavors to keep your protein intake enjoyable.

Healthy Fats: While moderation is key, healthy fats are an integral part of a balanced diet. Avocados, nuts, seeds, and olive oil offer a rich array of nutrients, including omega-3 fatty acids, which support heart health and overall well-being. Use them in cooking, salads, or as a satisfying snack.

Meal Timing for Maximum Effect

Beyond the content of your meals, the timing of your eating plays a pivotal role in optimizing metabolism and energy levels. Consider adopting a structured eating schedule that includes smaller, well-balanced meals throughout the day. This approach helps stave off excessive hunger, preventing overeating during main meals.

Strategic meal timing also involves exploring the concept of intermittent fasting, a practice that has gained traction for its potential benefits in weight loss and metabolic health. By designating specific windows for eating and fasting, you may enhance your body's ability to burn fat and regulate insulin levels.

As we navigate through the subtleties of creating a strategic meal plan, it's crucial to view this not as a restrictive diet but as a sustainable lifestyle change.

The objective is not merely to curb calories but to nourish your body with the right blend of nutrients, fostering habits that align with your rapid weight loss objectives. Stay tuned for practical tips, delicious recipes, and insightful strategies that will empower you on your journey to a healthier, more vibrant you.

Chapter Three

Hydration and Detoxification: Unlocking the Potential of Water for Weight Loss

In our ongoing quest for rapid weight loss, the seemingly simple yet profoundly impactful elements of hydration and detoxification come under the spotlight. This chapter aims to unravel the intricate relationship between optimal water intake and effective weight loss, delving into the physiological mechanisms that make water an indispensable ally in our pursuit of a healthier and more vibrant self. Additionally, we'll explore the concept of detoxification, investigating how certain beverages and herbal infusions can contribute to the cleansing of our internal systems.

The Importance of Water in Weight Loss

Water, often taken for granted in its simplicity, is a dynamic player in the weight loss game, influencing various physiological processes. Beyond its primary function of quenching thirst, adequate water intake is linked to a boosted metabolism, improved digestion, and enhanced calorie-burning capacity. Studies have suggested that consuming a glass of water before meals may promote a sense of fullness, potentially reducing overall calorie intake—a simple yet effective strategy.

Moreover, staying well-hydrated is paramount for optimal physical performance during exercise. Dehydration can lead to fatigue, impairing workout effectiveness and hindering overall progress. This chapter will not only emphasize the importance of consistent hydration but will also provide practical strategies to ensure you meet your daily water intake needs, making hydration an integral and strategic component of your weight loss plan.

Detoxifying Your Body

Detoxification, a concept often surrounded by a plethora of cleanses and diets, is explored here with a focus on natural and sustainable approaches. While extreme detox plans may lack scientific support and prove challenging to maintain, incorporating certain foods with detoxifying properties into your diet can support your body's innate cleansing mechanisms.

Antioxidant-rich foods, such as berries, leafy greens, and cruciferous vegetables, play a pivotal role in neutralizing free radicals and supporting the liver's detoxifying functions. Furthermore, the age-old practice of consuming herbal teas and infusions is examined for its potential benefits in detoxification. Dandelion tea, green tea, and peppermint tea are among the beverages traditionally associated with aiding the body in its natural cleansing processes.

This chapter will delve into the nuanced science behind these approaches, providing you with a comprehensive understanding of how hydration and detoxification can synergistically contribute to your rapid weight loss goals. It's important to approach these concepts with a balanced perspective, recognizing that while water and certain beverages can undoubtedly play a supportive role, they are most effective when integrated into a comprehensive and sustainable lifestyle plan. Stay tuned for practical tips, hydration strategies, and insights into natural detoxification methods that align with your goals for rapid weight loss.

Chapter Four

Effective Exercise for Quick Results

In the pursuit of rapid weight loss, exercise emerges as a dynamic catalyst, propelling your journey towards a healthier and more resilient body. This chapter will dissect the world of effective exercises, providing you with insights into high-impact routines that optimize calorie burning, boost metabolism, and contribute to sustainable weight loss.

High-Intensity Interval Training (HIIT)

At the forefront of efficient exercise regimens for rapid weight loss is High-Intensity Interval Training, commonly known as HIIT. This approach involves alternating between short bursts of intense activity and periods of rest or lower-intensity exercise. The beauty of HIIT lies in its ability to elevate your heart rate, maximize calorie expenditure, and stimulate fat burning—all in a shorter timeframe compared to traditional steady-state cardio workouts.

This chapter will guide you through various HIIT exercises, from bodyweight circuits to cardio-intensive routines, allowing you to tailor your workout to your fitness level and preferences. We'll explore the science behind HIIT, emphasizing its post-exercise calorie burn, known as the afterburn effect, which can contribute to ongoing fat loss even after you've completed your workout.

Incorporating Cardiovascular Exercises

Cardiovascular exercises are indispensable when it comes to burning calories and shedding excess weight. Whether it's brisk walking, running, cycling, or dancing, these activities engage large muscle groups, elevate your heart rate, and contribute to overall cardiovascular health.

We'll delve into the art of crafting an effective cardio routine, striking a balance between endurance-building exercises and interval-based sessions. By incorporating variety into your cardiovascular workouts, you not only keep things interesting but also challenge your body in different ways, preventing plateaus and maximizing weight loss potential.

Strength Training for Toning

While cardiovascular exercises focus on burning calories, strength training plays a pivotal role in toning and sculpting your body. Contrary to common misconceptions, strength training doesn't necessarily bulk up muscles; instead, it helps build lean muscle mass, which, in turn, boosts metabolism and contributes to a more defined physique.

This chapter will introduce you to fundamental strength training exercises, utilizing both bodyweight and resistance training. We'll emphasize the importance of a balanced fitness routine that combines cardio and strength training for comprehensive and sustainable weight loss results.

As we navigate through the world of effective exercises, remember that the key lies not just in the intensity but also in consistency. Finding activities you enjoy and incorporating them into your routine can make the journey towards rapid weight loss not only effective but also enjoyable. Stay tuned for practical workout routines, tips for staying motivated, and insights into the transformative power of exercise on your path to a healthier you.

Chapter Five

Sleep and Stress Management

In the intricate tapestry of rapid weight loss, achieving a balance between sufficient, quality sleep and effective stress management becomes paramount. This chapter unravels the profound impact that sleep patterns and stress levels can have on your body weight and overall well-being, offering practical strategies to optimize both for enhanced weight loss results.

The Role of Sleep in Weight Loss

Quality sleep is often hailed as a cornerstone of good health, and its significance extends to the realm of weight management. Insufficient sleep can disrupt hormonal balance, leading to an increase in hunger hormones like ghrelin and a decrease in satiety hormones like leptin. The result? Increased cravings, potentially derailing your weight loss efforts.

This chapter will delve into the science of sleep and its intricate relationship with metabolism, exploring strategies to improve sleep hygiene and establish consistent sleep patterns. From creating a conducive sleep environment to adopting relaxation techniques, we'll guide you on the path to optimizing your sleep for more effective weight loss.

Techniques for Stress Reduction

The fast-paced nature of modern life often brings with it elevated stress levels, which can be a significant impediment to weight loss. Chronic stress triggers the release of cortisol, a hormone associated with increased abdominal fat. Learning to manage stress effectively is not only beneficial for mental well-being but also for maintaining a healthy body weight.

This chapter will introduce you to various stress management techniques, from mindfulness meditation and deep breathing exercises to engaging in activities that bring joy and relaxation. By incorporating stress reduction practices into your daily routine, you create a supportive environment for your weight loss journey, allowing your body to function optimally.

Mindful Practices for Overall Well-being

Mindful living extends beyond specific practices; it encompasses a holistic approach to how you engage with your daily life. Mindfulness encourages being present in the moment, making intentional choices, and fostering a positive relationship with food and exercise.

We'll explore the concept of mindful eating, emphasizing the importance of savoring each bite, recognizing hunger and fullness cues, and cultivating a healthy relationship with food. By integrating mindful practices into your lifestyle, you not only enhance the effectiveness of your weight loss efforts but also contribute to overall well-being.

As we navigate through the realms of sleep and stress management, remember that sustainable weight loss is a holistic journey. By nurturing your body with adequate sleep and adopting effective stress reduction strategies, you pave the way for not only rapid weight loss but also a healthier and more balanced life. Stay tuned for actionable tips, practical techniques, and insightful practices to integrate into your daily routine for optimal results.

Chapter Six

Supplements and Boosters

In the pursuit of rapid weight loss, the integration of supplements and natural boosters can serve as additional tools to support your efforts. This chapter will explore the role of supplements in aiding weight loss, provide insights into natural boosters, and offer guidance on incorporating these elements safely into your regimen.

Understanding the Role of Supplements

Supplements can complement a balanced diet by providing essential nutrients, filling potential gaps, and supporting specific aspects of weight loss. However, it's crucial to approach supplements with a discerning eye, recognizing that they are not a substitute for a nutritious diet and healthy lifestyle.

This chapter will delve into popular weight loss supplements, examining the evidence behind their efficacy and potential risks. From vitamins and minerals to specialized supplements like green tea extract and garcinia cambogia, we'll guide you in making informed choices that align with your rapid weight loss goals.

Natural Weight Loss Boosters

Nature offers a myriad of compounds that may naturally support weight loss. From metabolism-boosting spices to herbs with potential fat-burning properties, incorporating these elements into your diet can provide additional support on your journey.

We'll explore the benefits of ingredients like green tea, cinnamon, and cayenne pepper, shedding light on how they may contribute to increased calorie burning and enhanced metabolism. Understanding the science behind these natural boosters empowers you to make intentional choices that align with your overall wellness goals.

Potential Risks and Precautions

While supplements and natural boosters can be beneficial, it's essential to be aware of potential risks and exercise caution. This chapter will outline common pitfalls, such as relying solely on supplements for weight loss or exceeding recommended dosages.

We'll provide guidance on choosing reputable supplements, understanding ingredient labels, and consulting with healthcare professionals before incorporating new elements into your regimen. Your health and safety are paramount, and a well-informed approach to supplementation is crucial for long-term success.

As we delve into the realm of supplements and natural boosters, remember that these elements are meant to enhance, not replace, a healthy lifestyle. By understanding their potential benefits and exercising caution, you can integrate them into your rapid weight loss plan as supportive tools. Stay tuned for practical tips, evidence-based insights, and a balanced perspective on navigating the world of supplements and boosters.

Chapter Seven

Tracking Progress and Adjusting Your Plan

Embarking on a journey of rapid weight loss requires a vigilant approach to tracking progress and making necessary adjustments along the way. This chapter delves into the importance of setting measurable goals, monitoring weight loss effectively, and adapting your plan to ensure sustained success.

Setting Measurable Goals

Clear and measurable goals provide a roadmap for your weight loss journey. This chapter will guide you through the process of setting realistic and achievable objectives, whether it's a specific target weight, inches lost, or improvements in overall fitness.

We'll explore the SMART criteria for goal setting—making goals Specific, Measurable, Achievable,

Relevant, and Time-bound. This framework ensures that your objectives are well-defined and aligned with your rapid weight loss timeline.

Monitoring Weight Loss

Regular monitoring of your progress is key to staying on track and making informed decisions about your weight loss plan. We'll discuss various methods of tracking, from regular weigh-ins to body measurements and visual assessments.

Understanding the concept of non-scale victories, such as increased energy levels, improved sleep, or enhanced mood, is integral to recognizing the holistic impact of your efforts. This chapter emphasizes a balanced approach to monitoring that goes beyond just the numbers on the scale.

Adjusting Your Plan for Long-Term Success

Flexibility is a crucial component of any successful weight loss strategy. As you progress, your body's needs may change, and adjustments to your plan may become necessary. This chapter provides insights into recognizing signs that modifications are needed and how to adapt your diet and exercise routine accordingly.

We'll discuss plateaus and how to overcome them, ensuring that you stay motivated and continue making progress. The goal is not just rapid weight loss in the short term but establishing habits that contribute to long-term success and a healthier lifestyle.

By the end of this chapter, you'll be equipped with the tools to assess your progress, celebrate achievements, and make informed adjustments to your plan. Remember, the journey to rapid weight loss is dynamic, and a willingness to adapt and learn from your experiences is essential for lasting success. Stay tuned for practical strategies, goal-setting techniques, and insights into maintaining momentum on your transformative path.

Chapter Eight

Maintaining a Healthy Lifestyle Beyond the Days

As your journey towards rapid weight loss nears its culmination, the focus shifts towards sustaining the progress you've achieved. This final chapter explores the transition from intense weight loss efforts to a balanced, long-term lifestyle that promotes both physical and mental well-being.

Transitioning to a Sustainable Diet

Sustainability is the key to maintaining your hard-earned weight loss. In this section, we'll discuss how to transition from a more restrictive diet to a sustainable eating plan. Emphasis will be placed on incorporating a variety of nutrient-dense foods, enjoying occasional treats in moderation, and cultivating a positive relationship with food.

We'll explore the concept of intuitive eating, where you listen to your body's cues and respond to hunger and fullness signals. This approach fosters a mindful and balanced relationship with food, making it easier to maintain a healthy weight over the long term.

Incorporating Regular Exercise

While the intensity of your workout routine during rapid weight loss may have been higher, it's essential to establish a long-term exercise plan that aligns with your lifestyle. We'll discuss how to transition from more intense workouts to sustainable forms of exercise that you genuinely enjoy.

Finding activities that bring joy and incorporating them into your routine will make exercise a sustainable and fulfilling part of your life. Whether it's walking, cycling, dancing, or engaging in recreational sports, the key is to stay active in a way that brings you genuine pleasure.

Building Long-Term Habits for Weight Maintenance

The final phase of your rapid weight loss journey is about solidifying the habits that contribute to weight maintenance. We'll discuss the importance of consistency, self-compassion, and resilience in the face of challenges.

This chapter will provide insights into creating a supportive environment that reinforces your healthy habits. From meal prepping and planning to cultivating a positive mindset, you'll gain practical strategies to navigate the nuances of maintaining your weight loss achievements.

Conclusion

Celebrating Achievements and Embracing a Healthier Lifestyle

As you conclude this transformative journey, take a moment to celebrate your achievements. Recognize the dedication and effort you've invested in your well-being. The conclusion will emphasize the importance of embracing a healthier lifestyle beyond the days of intense weight loss, understanding that the journey is ongoing, and self-care remains a lifelong commitment.

This final chapter encapsulates the essence of transitioning from rapid weight loss to a sustainable, healthy lifestyle—a journey that extends far beyond mere days and sets the stage for a vibrant, fulfilling life. Congratulations on your accomplishments, and may this chapter serve as a guide to a future filled with wellness and vitality.

www.ingramcontent.com/pod-product-compliance
Lightning Source LLC
Chambersburg PA
CBHW071003260726

48661CB00007B/2775